I'm Just Me- With a Food Allergy!

Written by Kathy Wormhood
with Katey Bellwood

To Grayson Thomas
And all allergy sufferers

This book began as an idea to educate school aged children.

Katey saw the need first-hand as the mother of a young child suffering with a severe peanut allergy.

As a social worker at an elementary school she realized that other children, as well as teachers, did not understand the severity of such an allergy.

This book was written to educate both children and adults on the various food allergies that plague our country.

As a grandmother, it has been difficult to see my grandson suffer and to watch my daughter try to cope while searching for answers and solutions.

We hope this book shines a light on a common, yet scary condition.

Many children have allergies to certain
foods or drink
That means when they
get near these things
They have to stop and think
These foods can hurt their bodies
Like make them sick or have a rash
This book will help you understand
Food allergies in a flash!

There are lots of kids who cannot eat

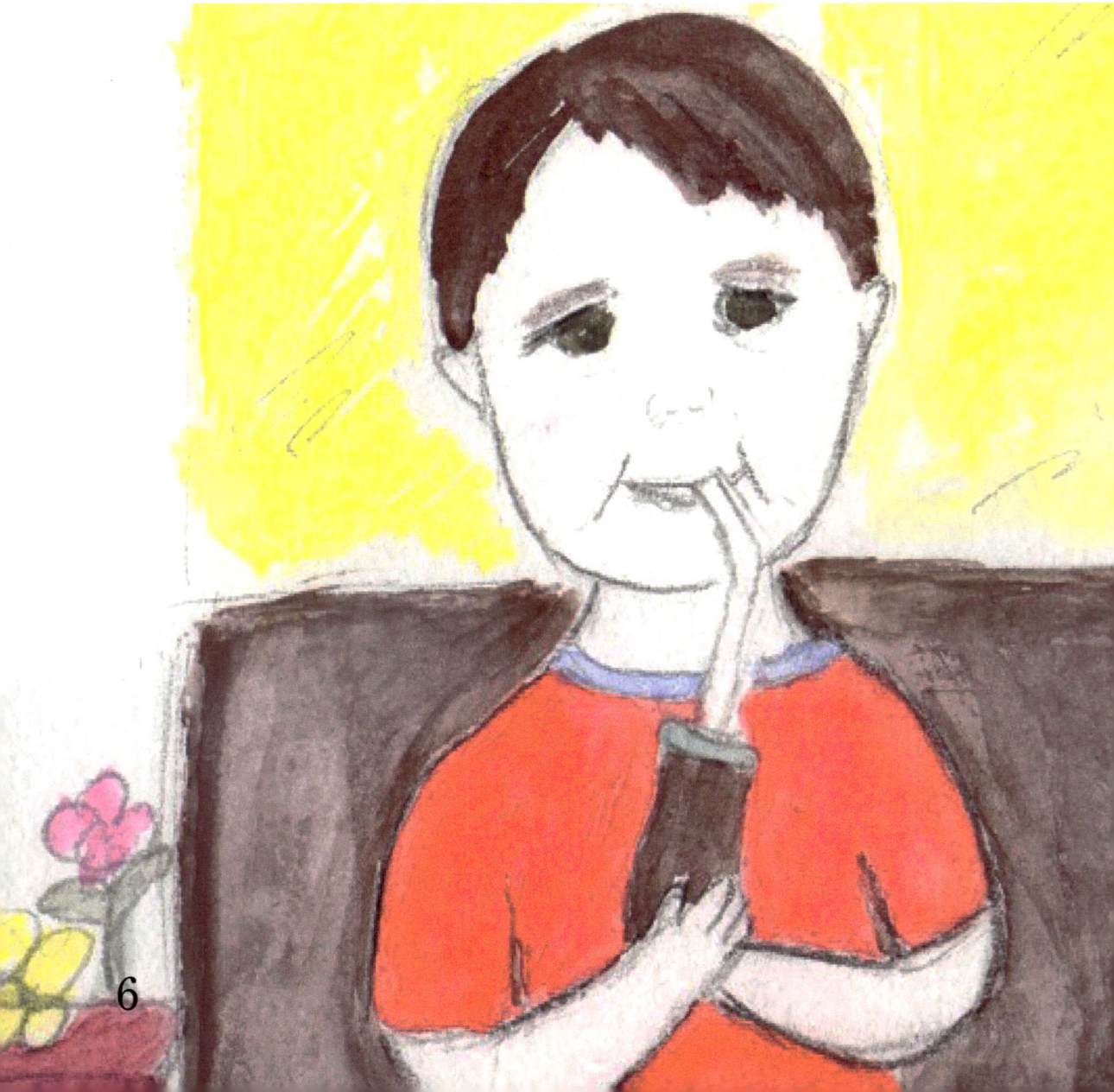

6

The same foods others do

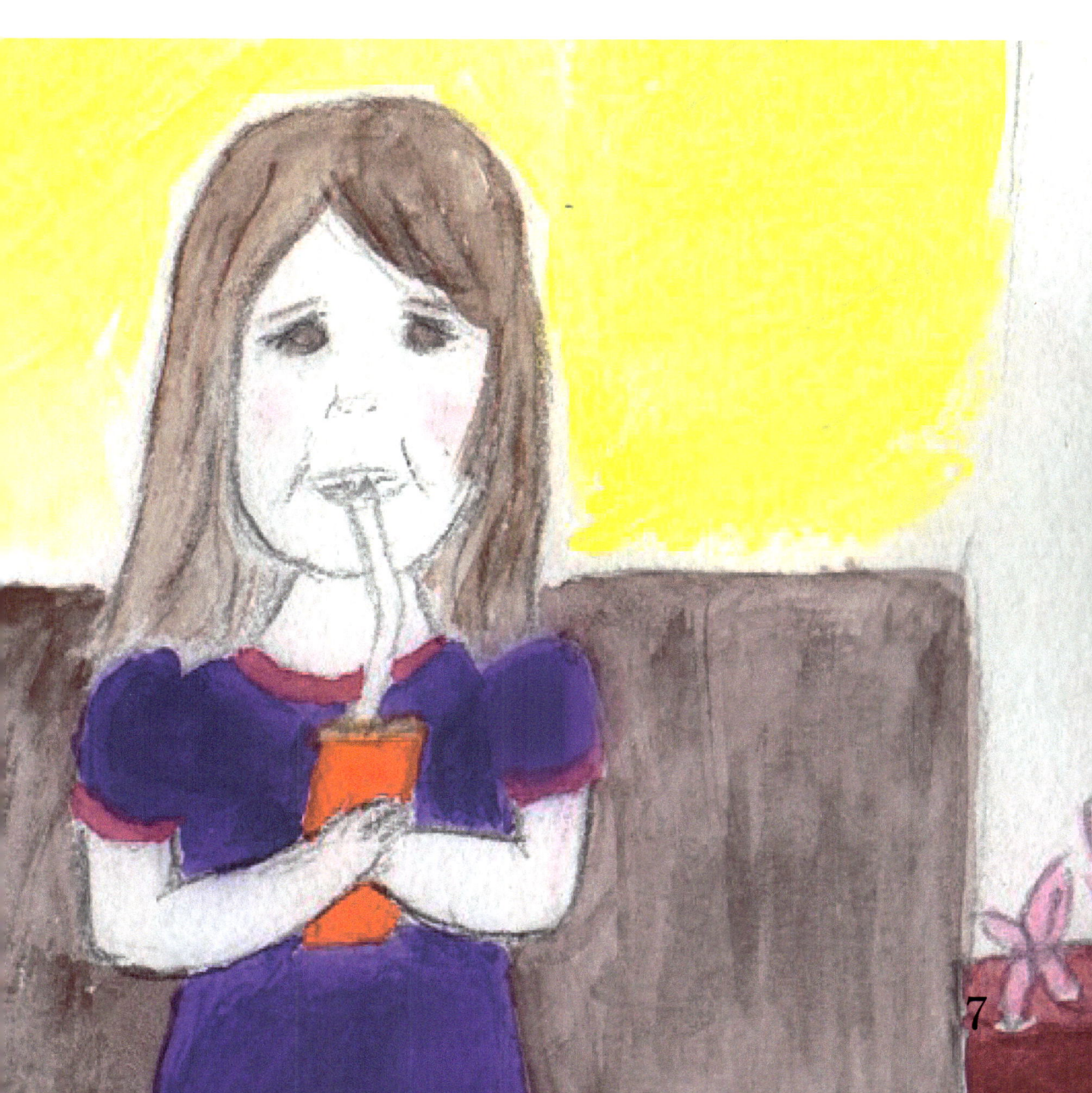

Different things
cause their belly
to hurt
Or makes them
have to poo!

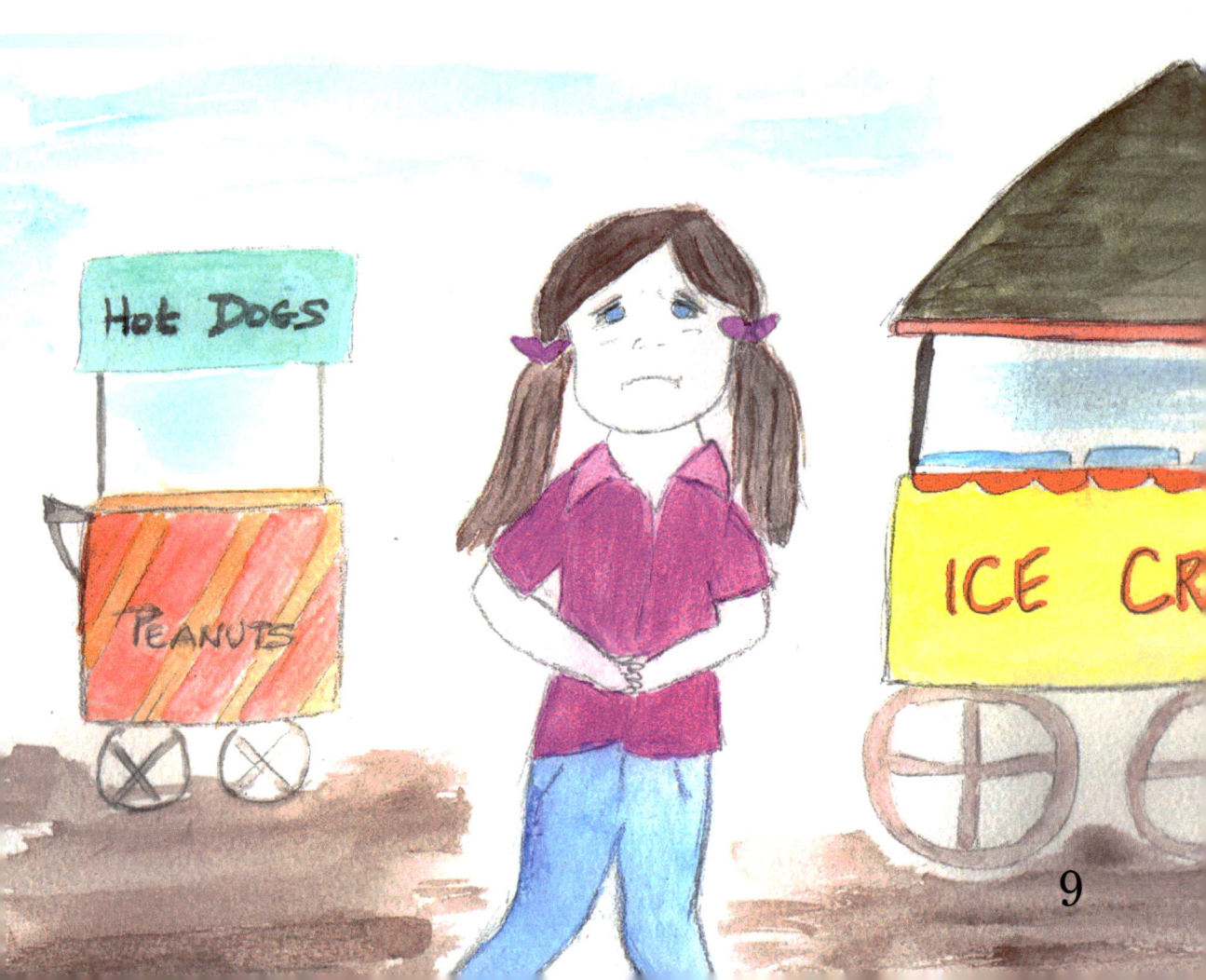

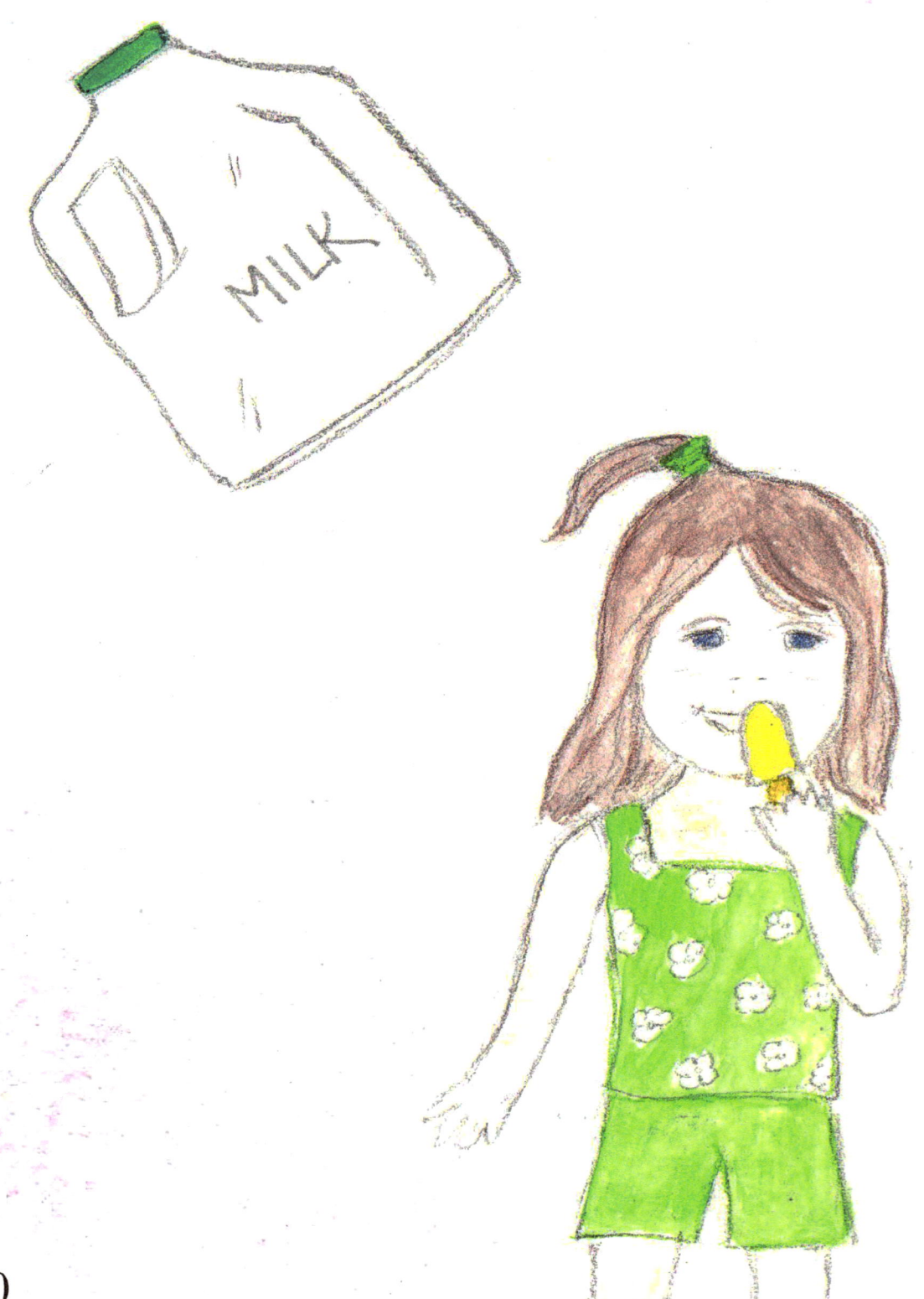

Like drinking milk or eating ice cream, tastes good to most kids I know.

But when I drink a milk shake or eat an ice cream cone

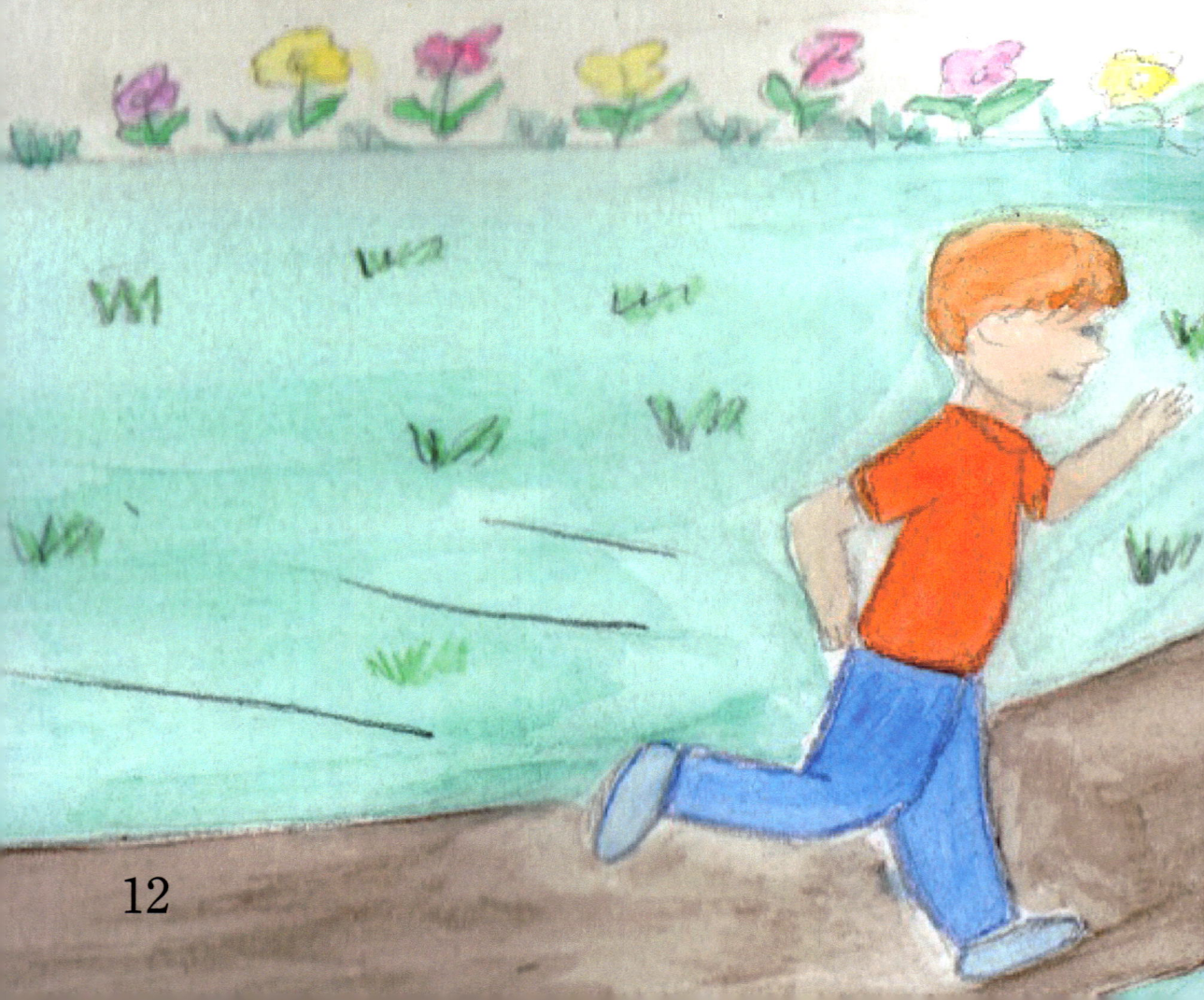

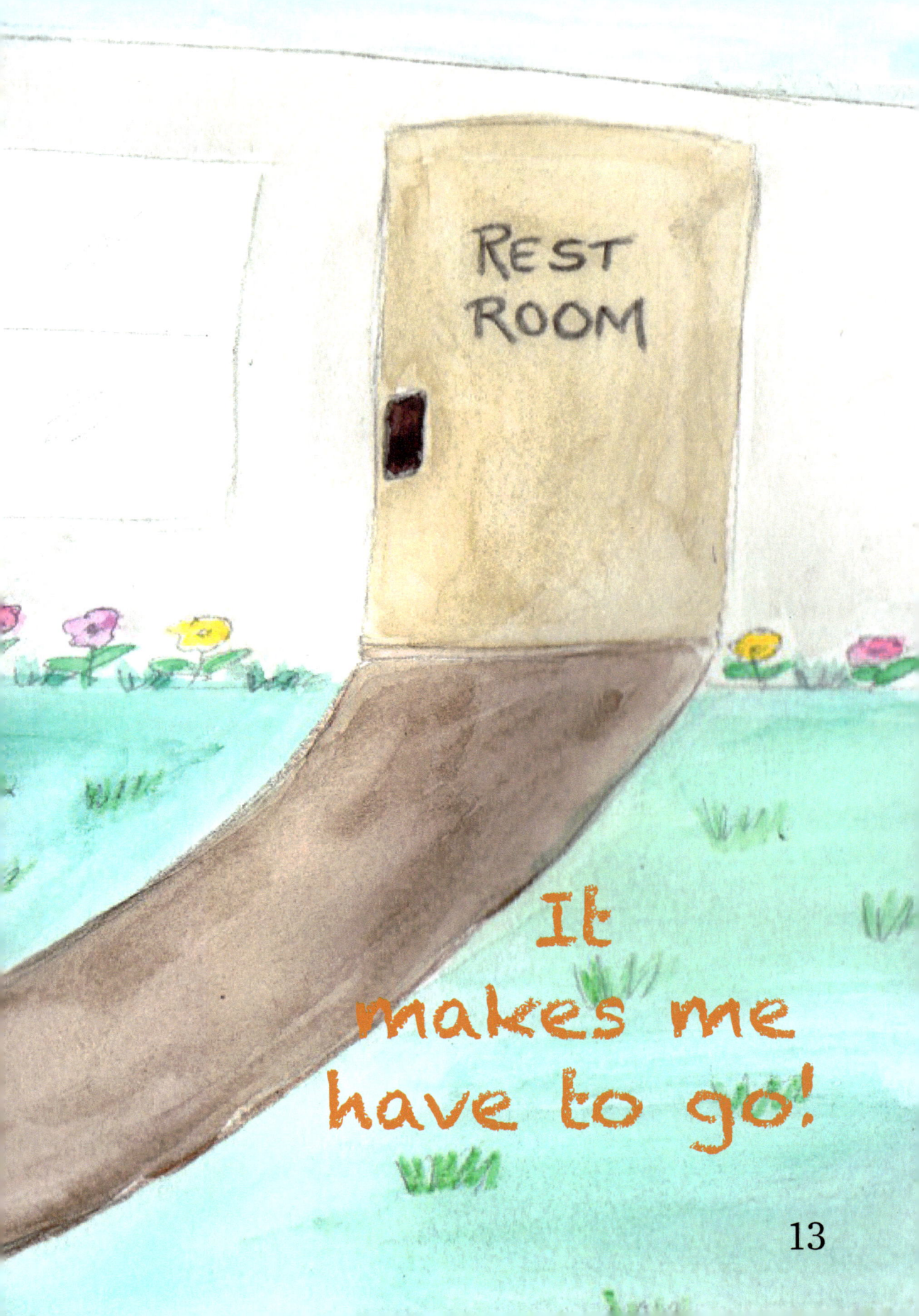

It makes me have to go!

Some kids cannot have anything with nuts

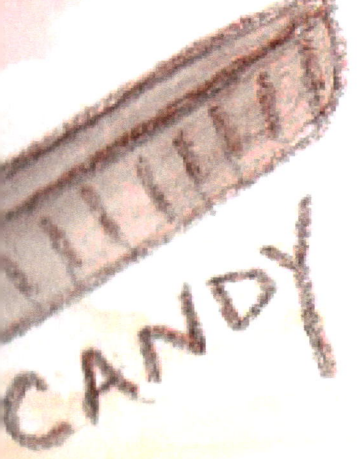

CANDY

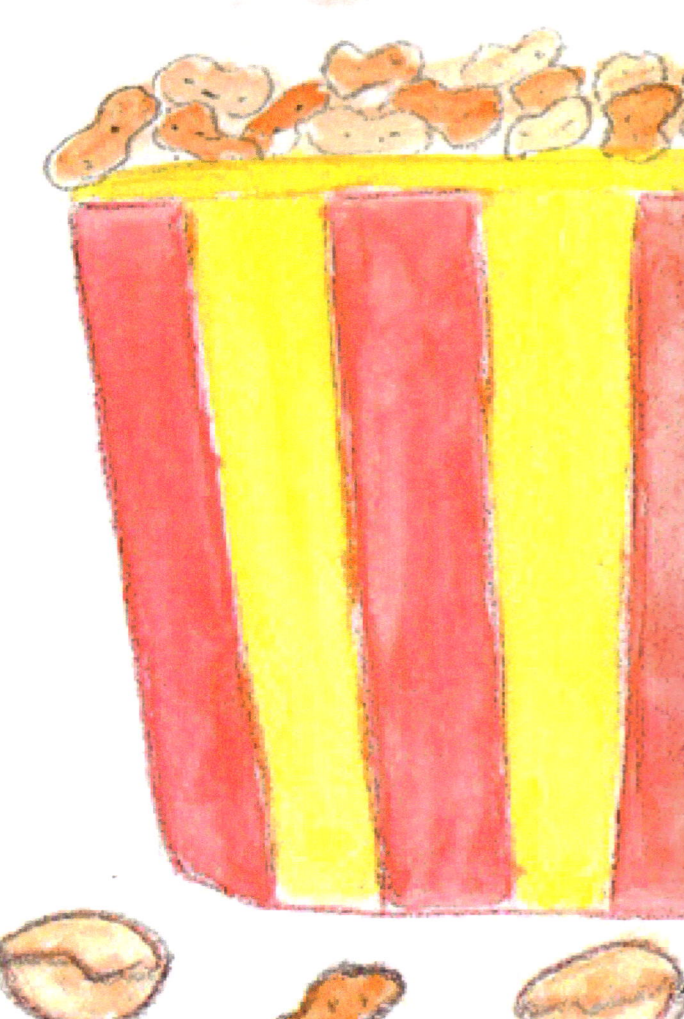

It makes their tongue feel funny

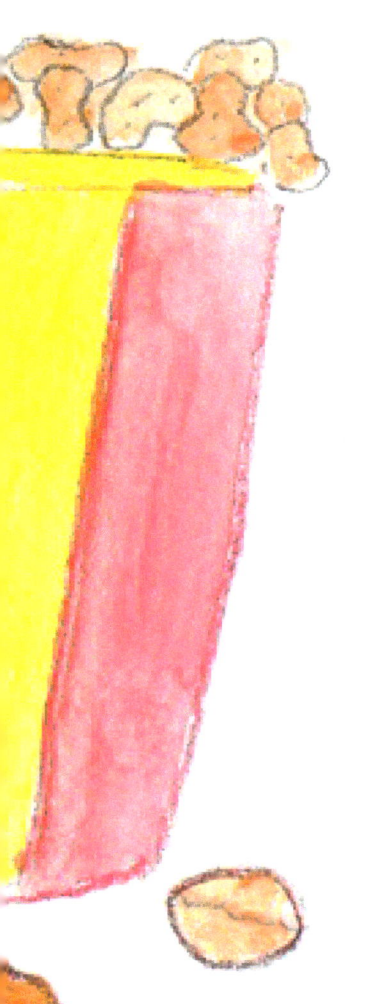

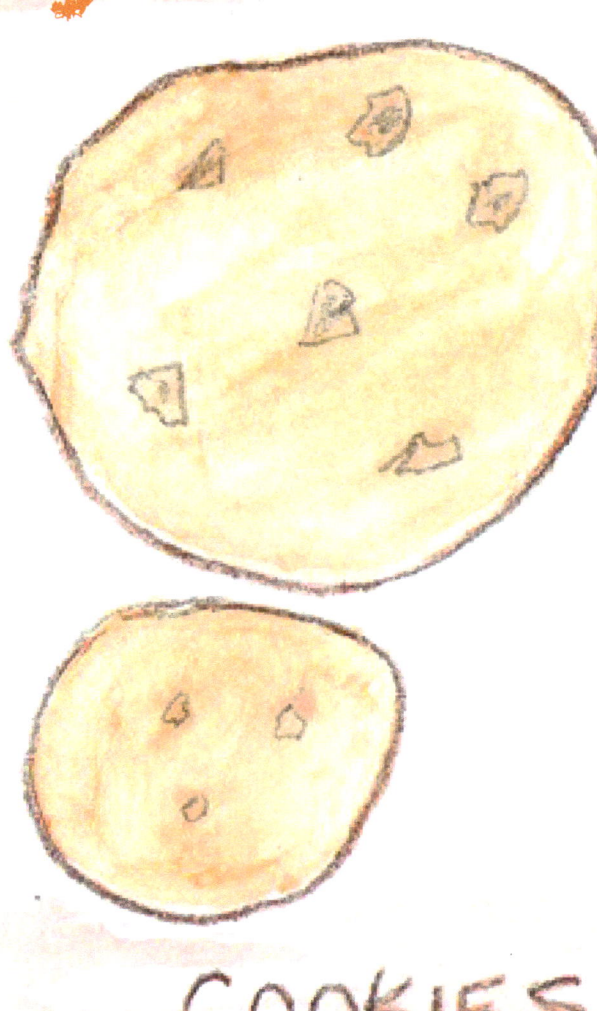

COOKIES

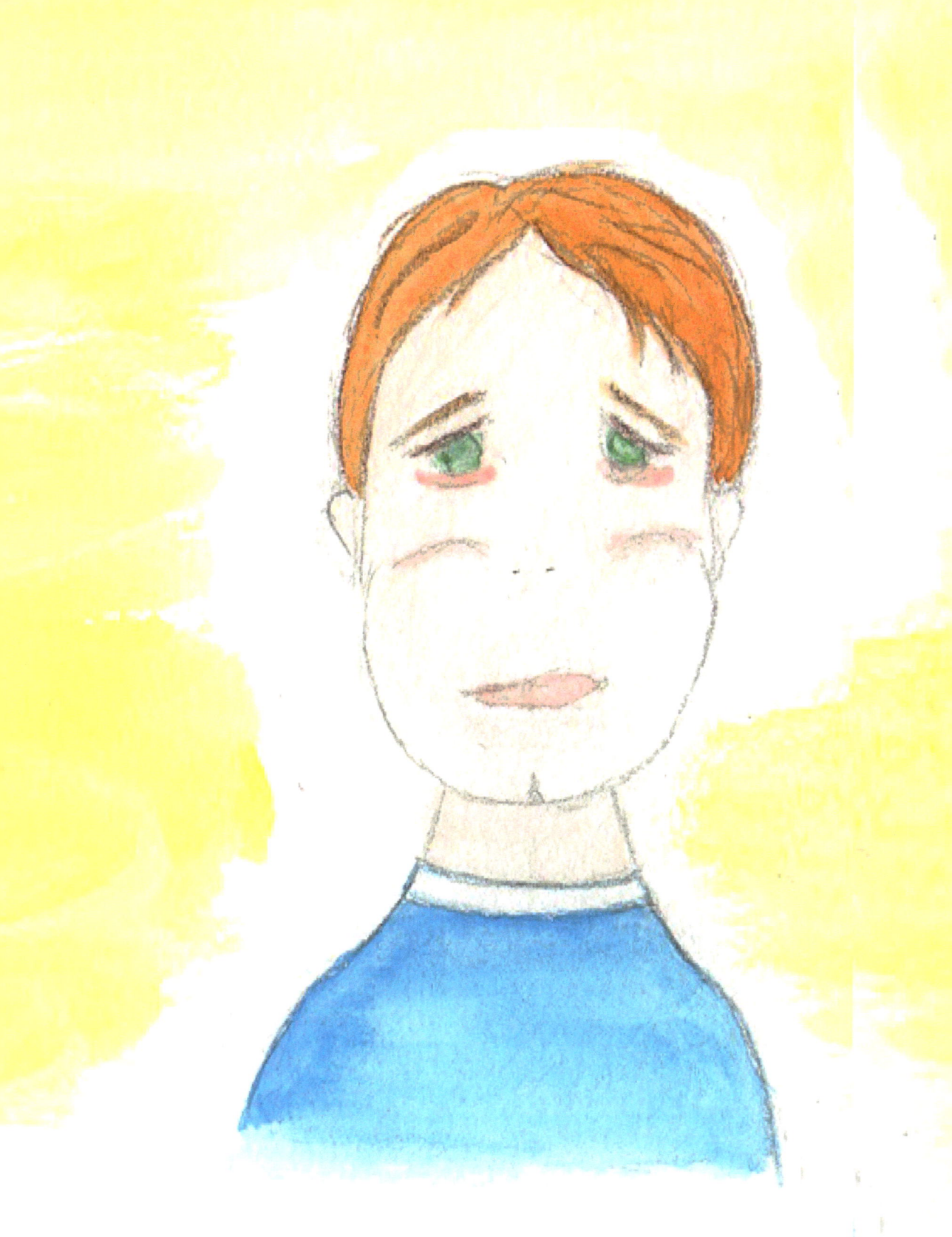

16

Their eyes get
red
Their lips may
swell
And their nose
will get all
runny.

When kids eat their sandwiches at lunch

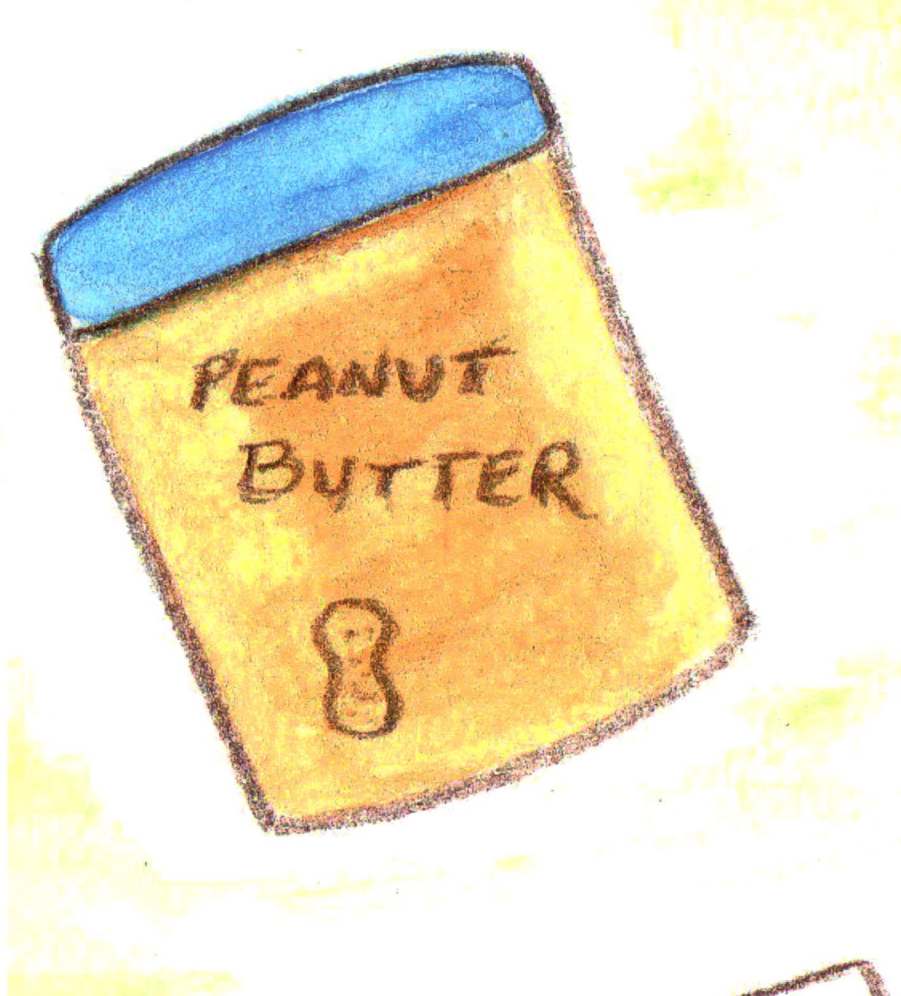

Especially peanut butter and jelly

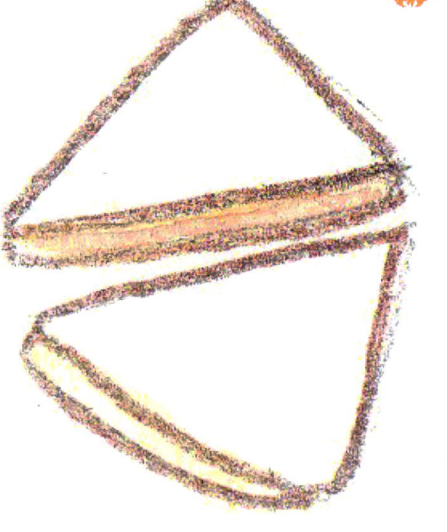

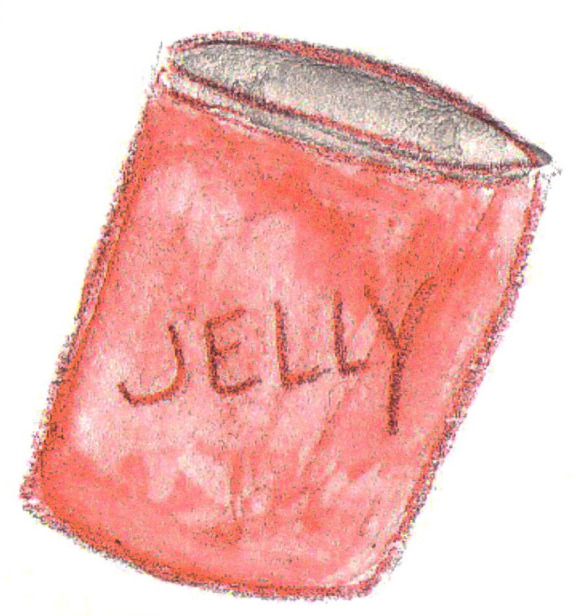

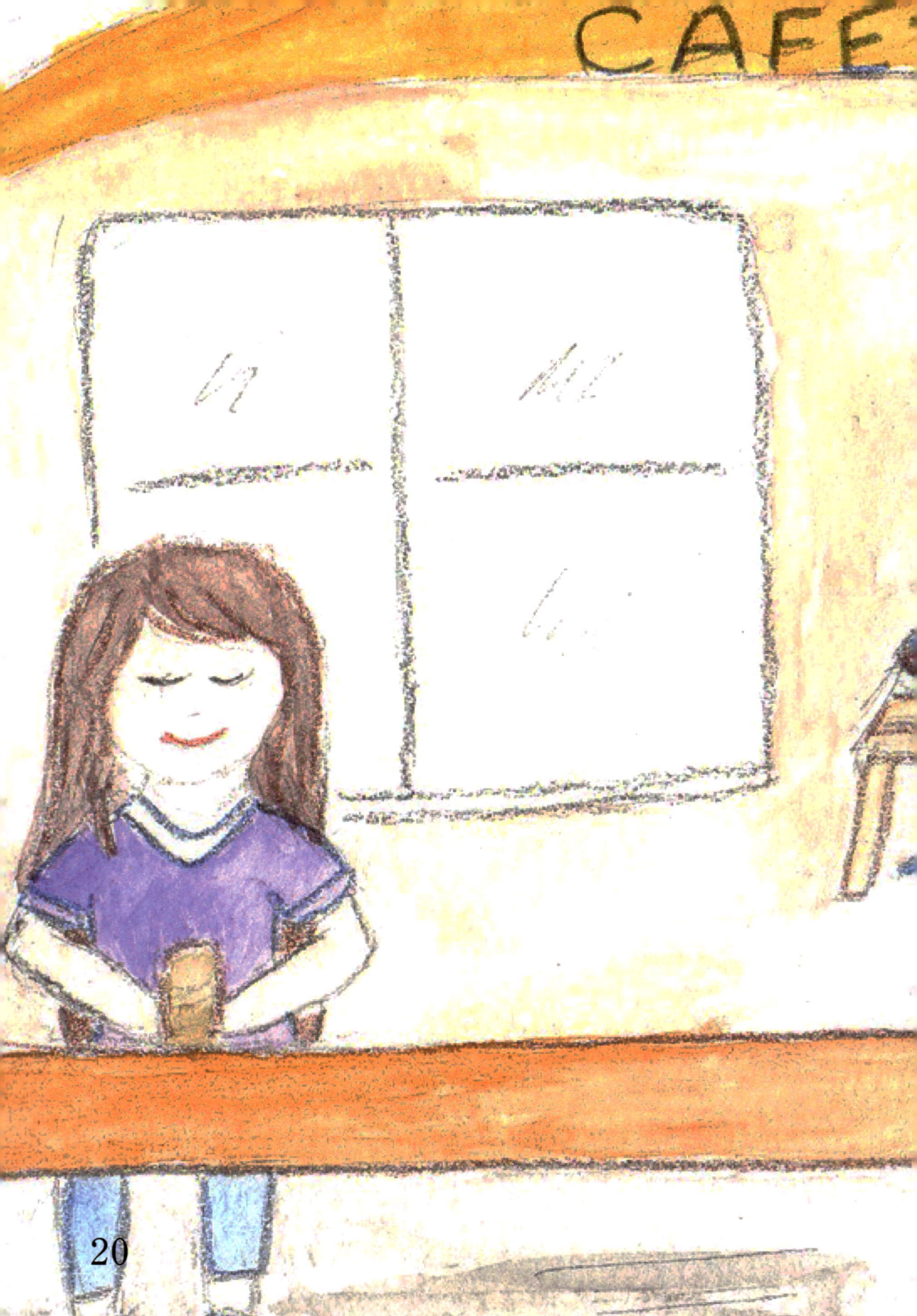

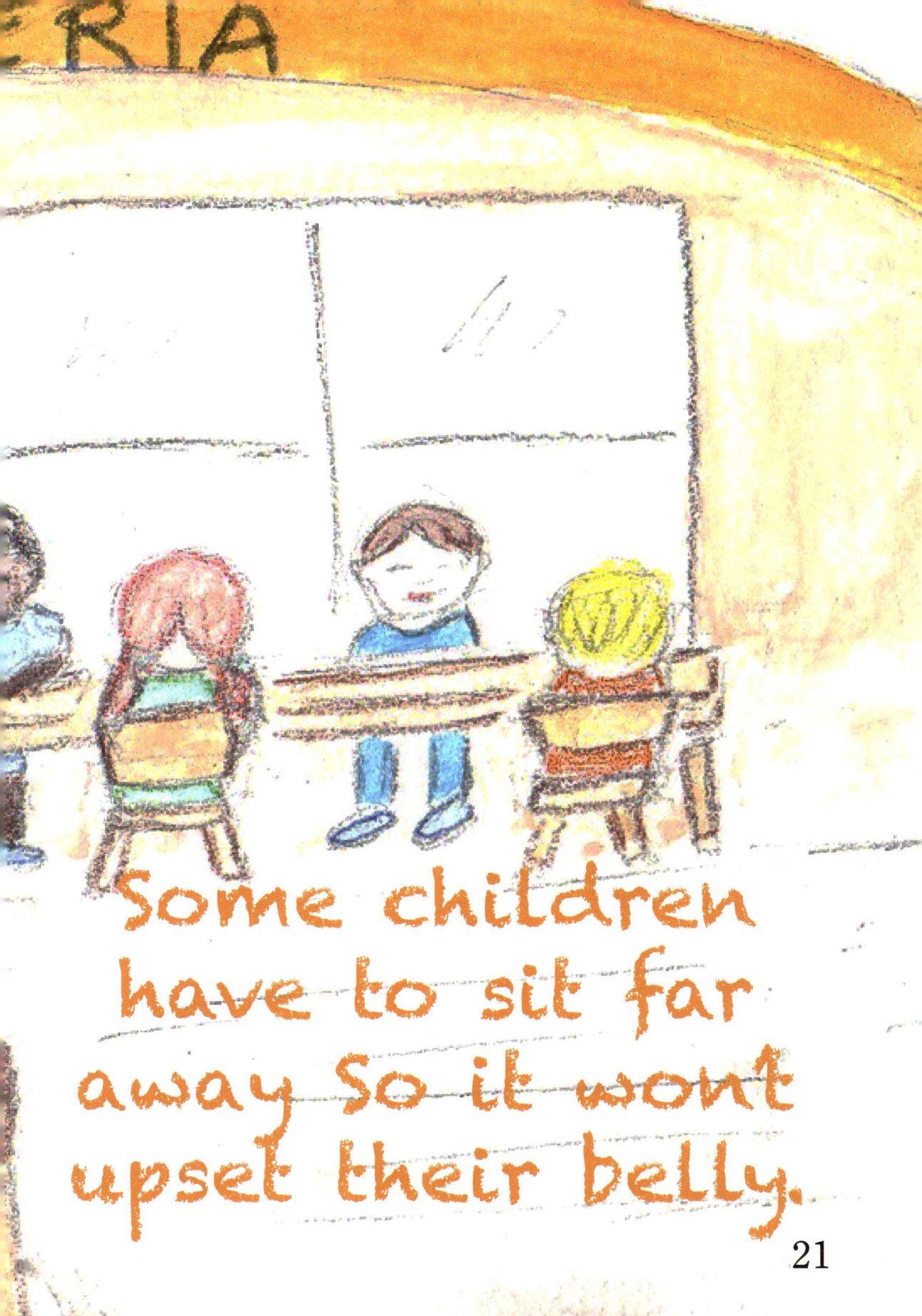

Some children have to sit far away so it wont upset their belly.

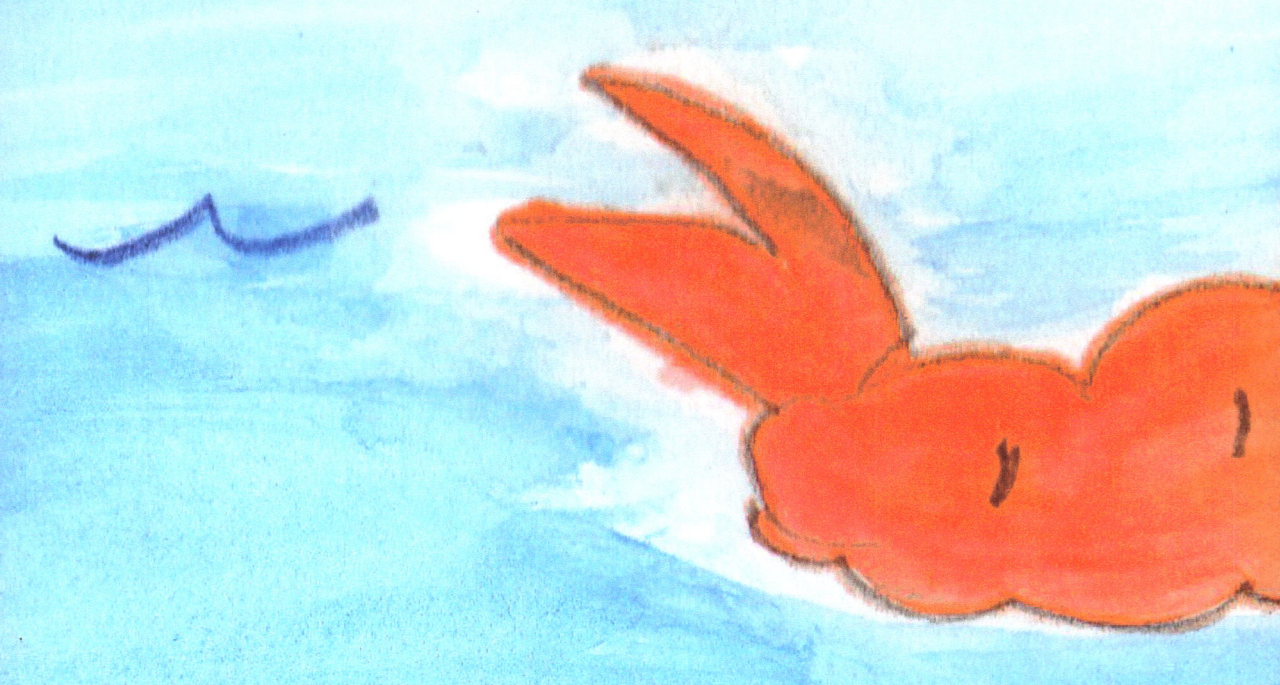

Although some
people eat
shellfish and
shrimp
For others it's a
downright scare

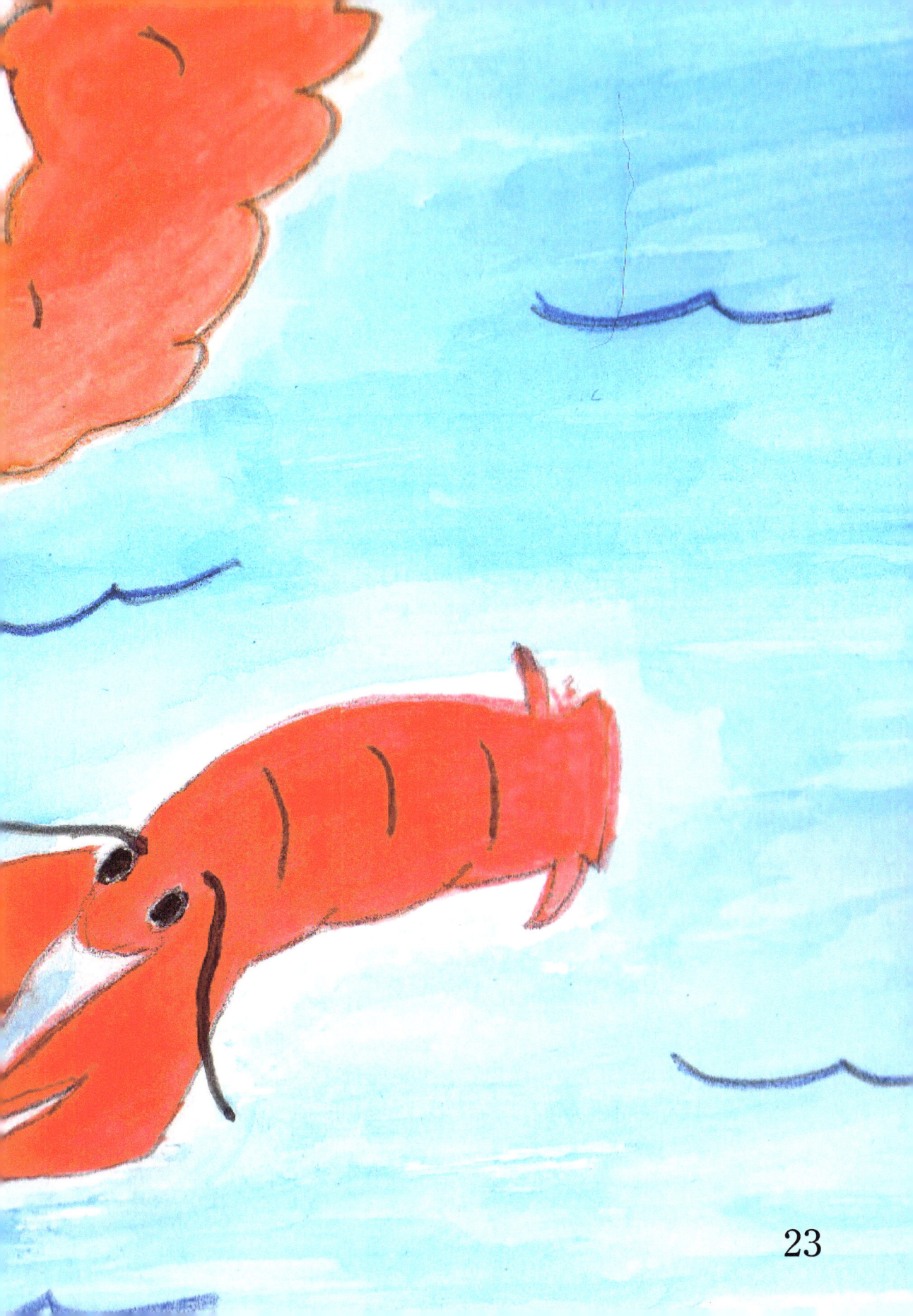

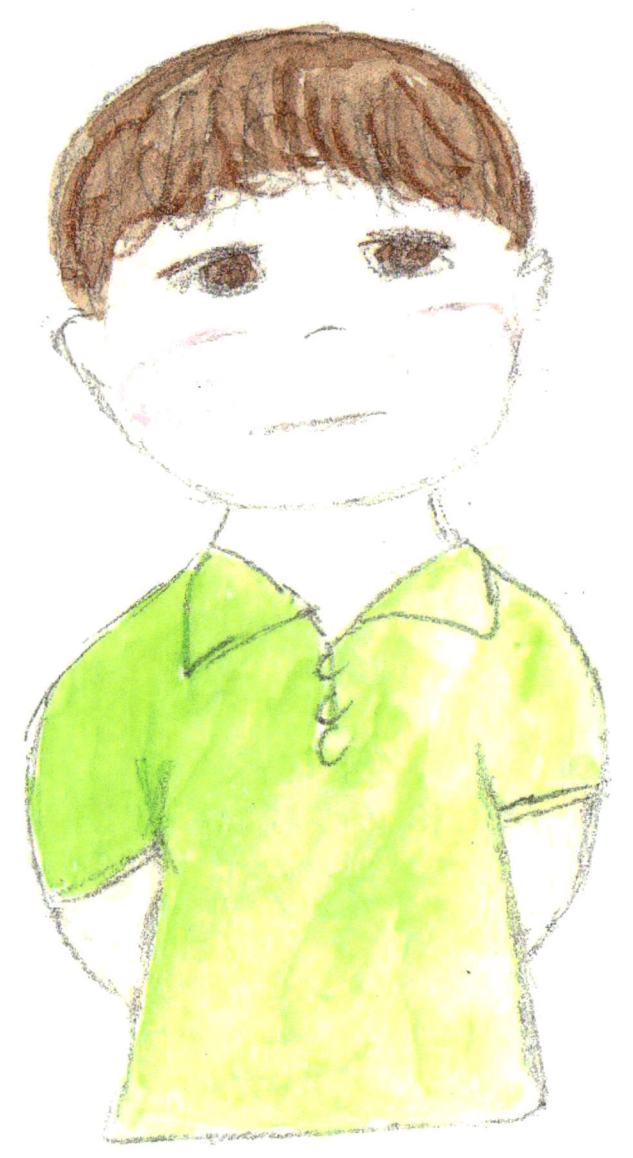

Their tummy
might churn
And their faces
may burn

They might even fall out of their chair!

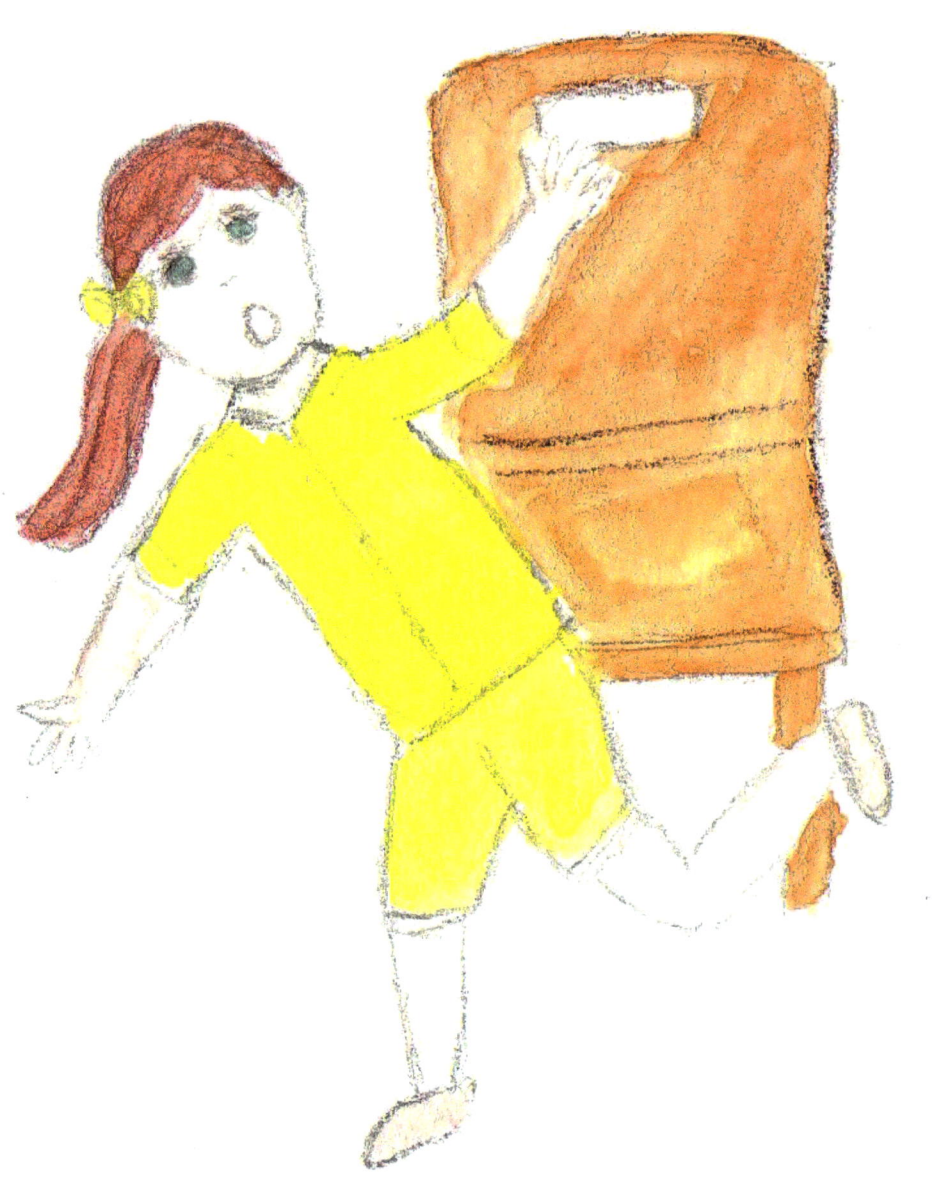

We can't help
that this happens
to us
If some foods
make us feel
icky

Our bodies are
not the same as
yours

And it can be
kind of tricky.

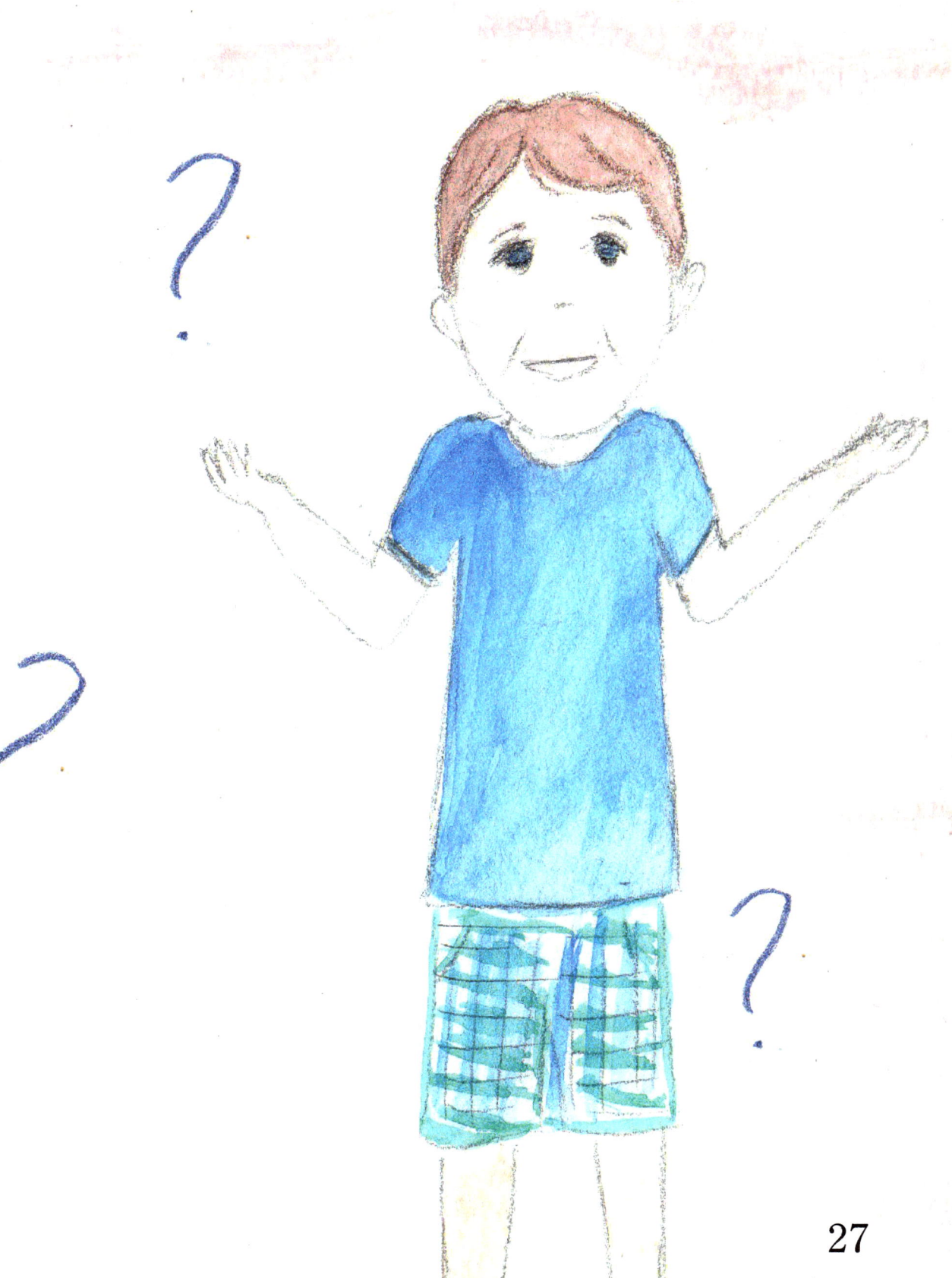

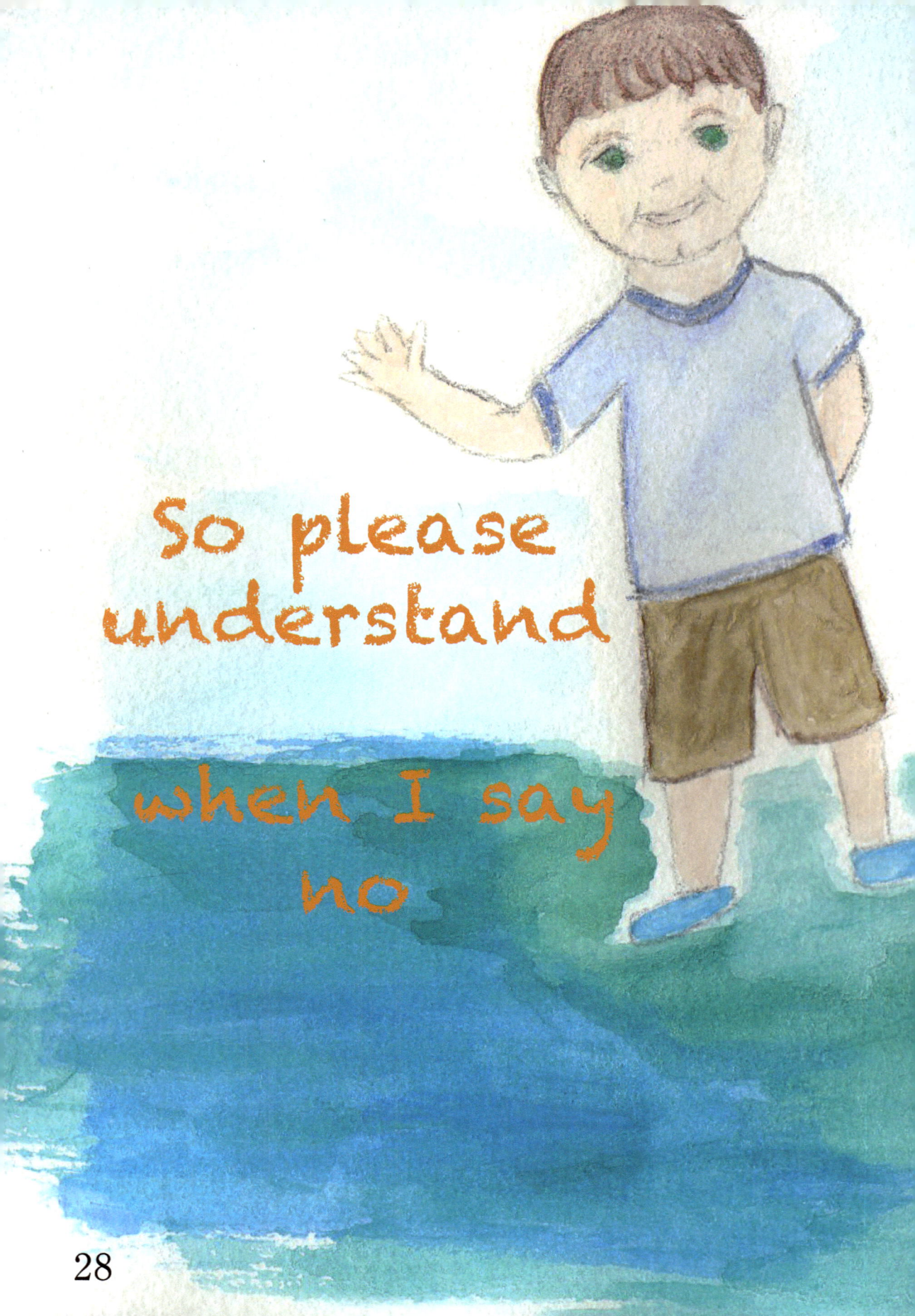

So please understand

when I say no

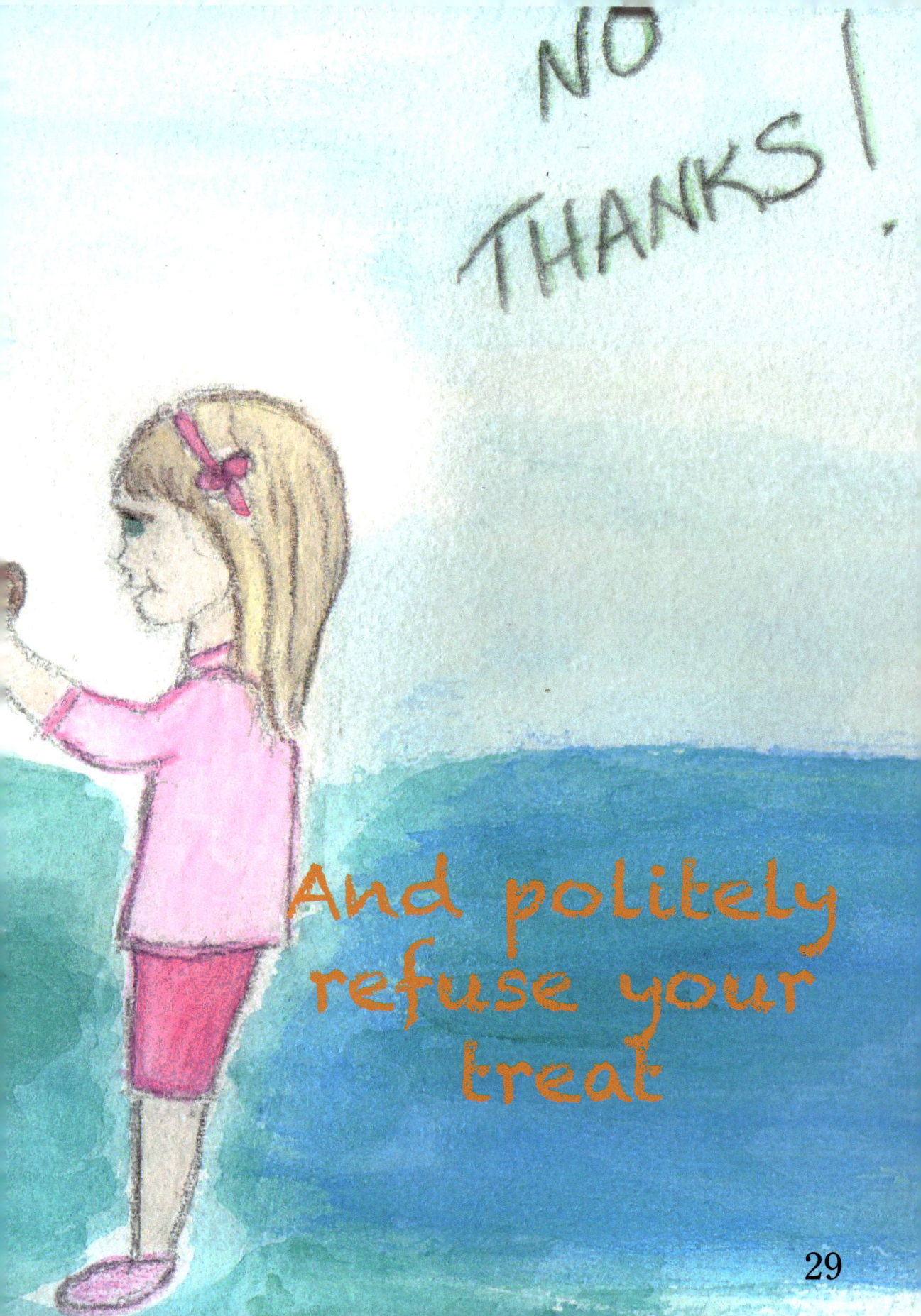

I'm not being
rude –
I just cant
have that food!

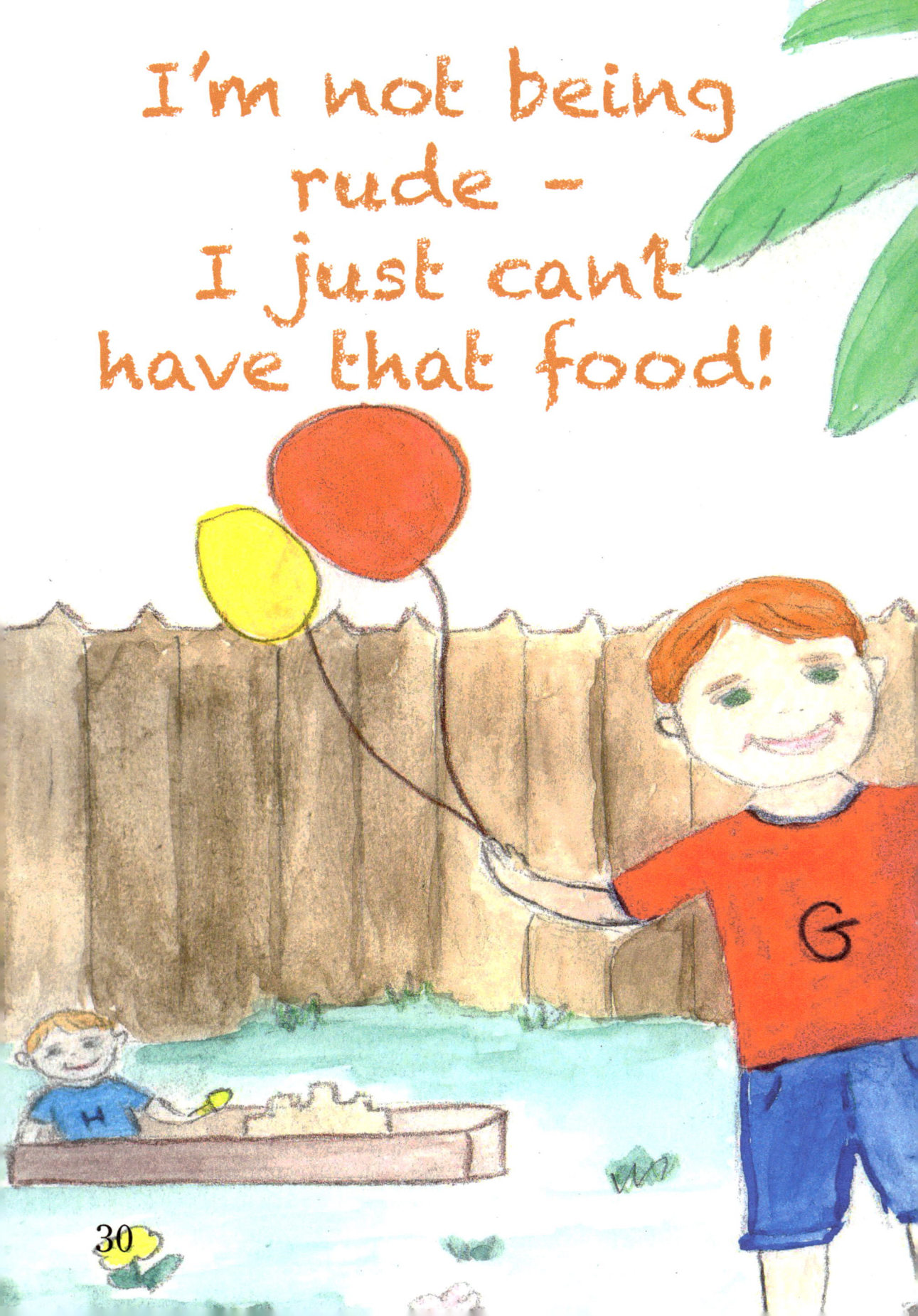

We can play
instead of
eat!

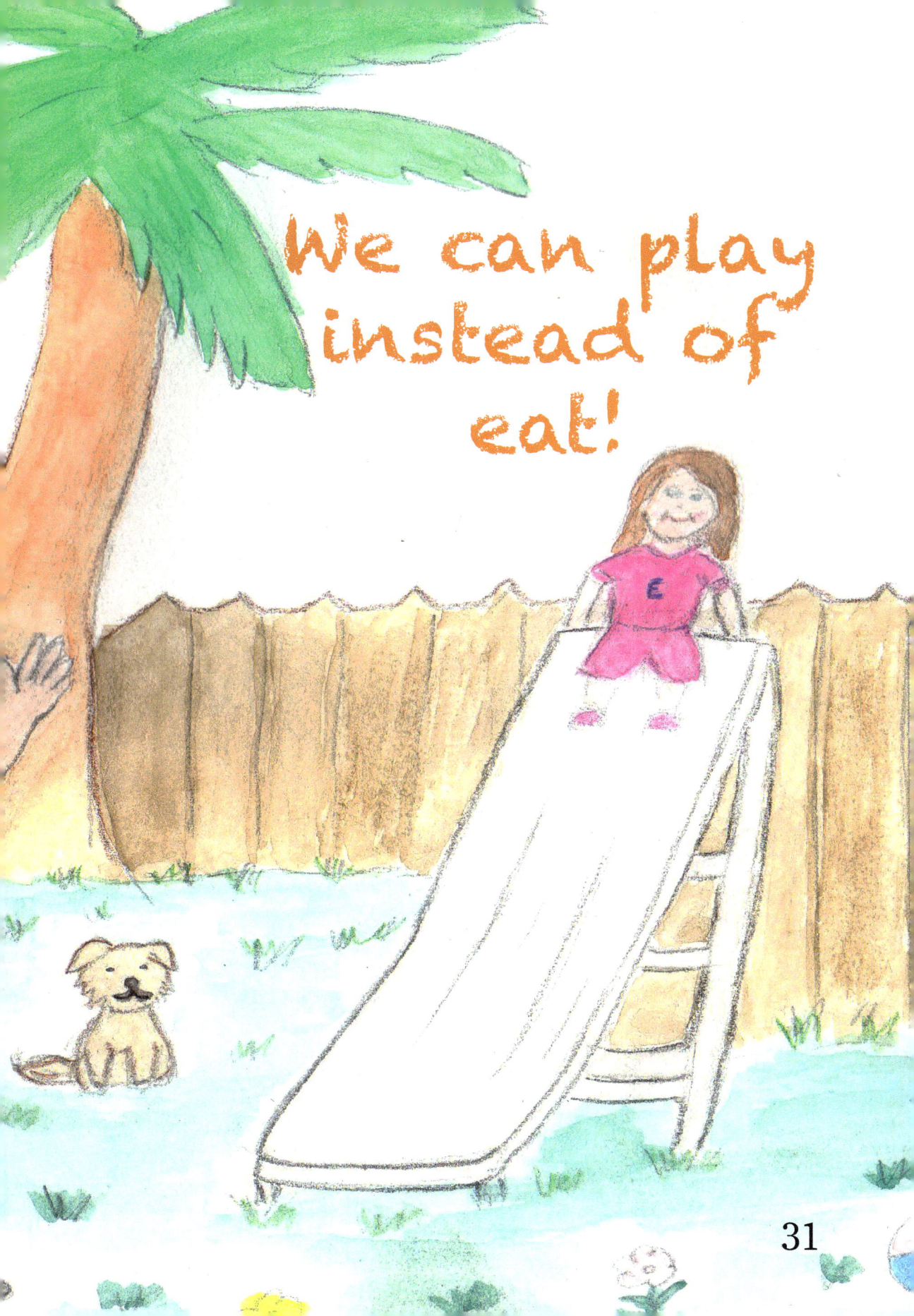

Thank you to Katey Bellwood for spreading the message for all food allergy sufferers.

Special thanks go to Amanda Sinni Photography and Hayley Livermore for their major contribution in putting this book together.

A big hug goes to Grayson, Emery and Hunter for being the perfect models needed for the artwork on this project.

Love you all,

Nana

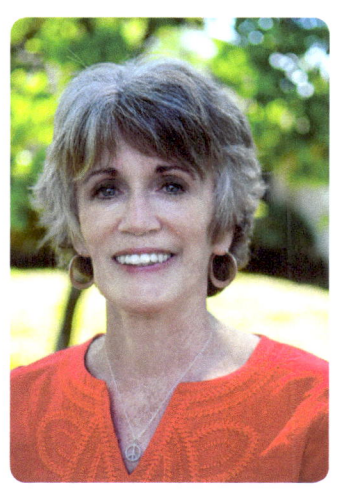

Kathy Wormhood is a writer of poetry, an illustrator and author of *Habits, Hosts and The Holy Ghost.*

I'm Just Me – With a Food Allergy is her first co-authored project.

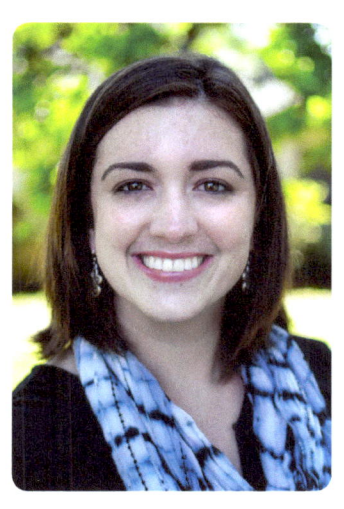

Katey Bellwood is a wife, mother and an elementary school social worker.

I'm Just Me – With a Food Allergy is her first published book.